Herbal Antibiotics For Beginners:

Treat, Heal, Prevent Illness and Resist Viral Infections

By

Brittany Samons

Table of Contents

Introduction 5

Part 1. Antibiotic Basics 6

Part 2. Natural Antibiotics 9

    Garlic 9

    Onion 12

    Aloe Vera 15

    Ginger 18

    Rosemary 21

    Sage 23

    Honey 26

    Cabbage 28

    Cinnamon 31

    Basil 33

Final Words 35

Thank You Page 36

Herbal Antibiotics For Beginners: Treat, Heal, Prevent Illness and Resist Viral Infections

By Brittany Samons

© Copyright 2015 Brittany Samons

Reproduction or translation of any part of this work beyond that permitted by section 107 or 108 of the 1976 United States Copyright Act without permission of the copyright owner is unlawful. Requests for permission or further information should be addressed to the author.

This publication is designed to provide accurate and authoritative information in regard to the subject matter covered. This work is sold with the understanding that the publisher is not engaged in rendering legal, accounting, or other professional services. If legal advice or other expert assistance is required, the services of a competent professional person should be sought.

First Published, 2015

Printed in the United States of America

Introduction

Herbal antibiotics have been around for centuries acting as natural healing agent in our bodies. They are used to ward off or to get rid of infections, flu, cold and sometimes major diseases too. They might be slow but they are safer and more reliable. They are extremely potent in fighting against the diseases, strengthening the immunity system and eradicating the stress caused by external factors.

There is a general approach that medicines are employed once an individual gets affected by a disease so why not strengthen the immunity beforehand to ensure safety from protection from the disease in the first place.

The answer to the safety and prevention of diseases lies in the fact that use of harmful medicines is avoided and herbal treatment is used which is a natural way of dealing with the issues. There are multiple types of natural antibiotics to fight against harmful bacteria.

The article envisages the use of 10 natural and herbal antibiotics that are useful to strengthen the immunity system and ensure a healthy life.

Part 1. Antibiotic Basics

What is antibiotic?

Antibiotic is also known as antibacterial. It is used to destroy or slow-down the growth of an infection caused by harmful bacteria. Antibiotic carefully attacks the bacterial cells to obliterate them and leave out the human cells unaffected. Some common harmful bacteria can cause illnesses such as tuberculosis, syphilis, meningitis and salmonella.

How do antibiotic work on our body?

If you think taking regular antibiotic drugs will help you fight illness, then you are mistaken. As per commons studies, it has been observed that people who take antibiotic medicines incessantly to ward-off infections get infected with diseases more frequently than people who take antibiotic occasionally. The idea is to create balance as excess antibiotic drugs can disturb your bodily function by destroying good bacteria as well. Now if you are wondering why this happens, it is because there are very few antibiotics that specifically target only bad bacteria. So, when conventional antibiotics are ingested, there are good bacteria that come in the way and get destroyed too. This creates more room for the bad perhaps more harmful bacteria in the body which is why antibiotics are to be ingested very carefully to maintain proper balance of the body. This varies from case to case as pharmaceutical antibiotics are of two kinds:

Bactericidal – Bactericidal is an antibiotic that kills harmful bacteria in the body

Bacteriostatic – Bacteriostatic is an antibiotic that prevents bacteria from multiplying

What are herbal antibiotics?

The term herbal comes from herbs and nature. Herbal antibiotics are mild, natural medicines used to regularize body's imbalance. But be aware, these herbs act differently on every person's body just like synthetic medicines. The only difference is that because herbal antibiotics are natural and come from nature, they won't do you any harm unlike pharmaceutical antibiotics. Herbal antibiotics are basically meant to build and strengthen the body's immune system without really causing any harm to the body. Some of these herbal antibiotics may also treat major illnesses but as mentioned above it may vary depending on the body type. Natural herbs can however be used in place of antibiotics to improve a body's function naturally.

How do herbal antibiotics work?

Herbal antibiotic is nature's gift to humans and since it's been around for years and centuries, the quality of antibiotic has evolved and so have the compounds present in these natural ingredients. These herbs contain countless active compounds that help the body heal naturally.

Part 2. Natural Antibiotics

Below are 10 natural antibiotic ingredients to help you stay healthy and disease-free.

Garlic

Garlic is one of the best and widely used herbs around the world. It is used as a flavouring agent in regular meals. However, not many are aware of what magic this little herbal clove can do. As per scientists, an experiment regarding garlic's antibacterial competency was conducted wherein the bacteria immediately died once it came in contact with fresh garlic. So do you see how strong this kitchen staple is? Other tests have also proved that garlic can easily kill at least 72 harmful bacteria in the body if consumed proportionally. Its presence in the kitchen renders its access easier and its ingestion via morning juice or in raw form can escalate the immunity strength to awe-inspiring levels where an individual would not only enjoy a life safe from all diseases but also perform better in his daily tasks.

Over the years, garlic's strong antibacterial properties have proved to treat serious conditions such as heart diseases, infected blood system, high blood pressure problem, high cholesterol, heart attacks and artery problems. This implies that in this current age where the use of junk food is dominant, this natural ingredient can suffice to address most of the issues associated to the heart. It acts as a counter strategy against the harmful effects of the prevalent junk food. Moreover, experts suggest that garlic naturally helps to slow down the development of atherosclerosis too.

Garlic has also been used to prevent many types of dangerous cancer such as rectal cancer, colon cancer, breast cancer, stomach cancer, lung cancer and prostate cancer.

The best thing about ingesting garlic is that unlike pharmaceutical antibiotic or other medicines, garlic does not destroy healthy bacteria in our body. More and more people these days are turning to this trustworthy kitchen item as it helps fight minor infections, cold, flu and sinus problems too. Many people also use garlic oil or garlic juice to treat external infections such as athletes foot, itch, fungal infection, warts and corns. Garlic has a compound called allicin. This is what majorly helps to eliminate bacteria.

How to ingest garlic as an antibiotic?

For best results, it is advised to ingest raw garlic. It is also good to eat fresh garlic than aged garlic as they are less effective on the bacteria. Experts suggest three to four cloves a day to maintain proper health as it helps the body to stay healthy both externally and internally.

Peel at least three to four cloves. Crush them and set these cloves in place for about 10 minutes. This process allows garlic to activate its germ killing compound by being exposed to the air. Have it with salad or perhaps add it to your morning vegetable juice.

Onion

You've seen many types of onions, many colors and sizes too. They are easily available and one of the most important ingredient when cooking food. Are we forgetting something? Yes! This genius vegetable is loaded with antibacterial and anti-fungal properties that help the body to fight against infections related to the respiratory tract, flu and kidney problem. Onion is also filled with sulphur-compounds that has a cleansing effect on the body and basically flushes out most harmful bacteria regularly that cause us to fall sick. Onions also helps treat or prevent cardiovascular disease. Unless you suffer from gastritis reflex, there is no reason you should not be taking full advantage of this nature's gift every single day. Onion must be a part of your daily diet and of course just like any other, it provides the best result when consumed raw.

In the ancient time, probably many centuries ago, the first ever antibiotic added in a pharmaceutical medicine was sulphur-compound and onions are loaded with this compound. Thus, it can be implied that the use of onion as an antibiotic is not effective but traditional as well. The authenticity and reliability of this natural ingredient cannot be further insisted by stating the fact that it is not only in use for a long time but it is also effective in producing results. The human race has been relying on it due to its positive results.

Onions are safe to be eaten every day, raw or cooked. However, be careful and only ingest a proportionate amount as onions are broad-spectrum antibiotics and can kill healthy bacteria too.

How to ingest onion as an antibiotic?

Onions are to be eaten raw to be effective on the bacteria and to build your immunity system. So, try adding a raw, medium sized onion to your regular salad along with other greens. Onion soup, onion added in other foods is always a plus. So, don't hold back and eat onion to stay healthy every day. As stated, the daily use can escalate the strength of the immunity system and who wouldn't take a few pieces of onion if it acts positively against the diseases and suppresses their occurrence.

Here's a simple recipe to treat sinus problem:

Chop an onion and toss it in a bowl. Place your head over the bowl and color your head with a towel. Inhale the fresh fragrance of onion for a few minutes and you will feel an instant relief from you sinus trouble.

Aloe Vera

Aloe vera plant is a member of Lily family. It is originally found in Africa but has had increased distributions lately throughout the world for not just the way it looks but because of its medicinal use in pharma companies and households. Aloe vera is loaded with vitamins, nutrients, minerals, enzymes amino acids and salicylic acid. Moreover, aloe vera is the only natural source of vitamin B12 in today's day and age. There are hormones in aloe vera that help speed up the healing process of the body.

Aloe vera juice is easily available in the market and this is also one of the liquids that are recommended by herbal doctors as it naturally helps balance the body's immune system to fight infections. Aloe vera has also proved to work as a helpful compound to get rid of stress and anxiety. So, all in all, aloe vera is the best replacement for anti-depressants or anti-anxiety drugs. Many patients swear by aloe vera juice and claim to have developed a calm attitude since consuming aloe vera juice. Many also claim that it has a soothing effect in the body and mind.

Health Benefits:

Aloe vera gel is the best remedy for people suffering from diabetes as they are prone to getting infections and ulcers especially in the foot area. Using aloe vera gel topically on the wound or infection not only soothes it but also heals it over time.

People with sensitive skin who are prone to sun burn can also use aloe vera gel to cool the skin down as the gel helps reduce the burning sensation instantly.

Aloe vera gel has been used by many to reduce scars caused by wounds, cuts and even acne. Aloe vera gel applied directly to the affected area on the regular helps decrease these scars.

Aloe vera juice helps strengthen the body's immune system naturally.

Applying aloe vera gel on wounds and infections eases the pain whilst eradicating the bacteria.

Thus, it can be concluded that Aloe Vera is really useful in eradicating the injuries, bringing the glow and freshness to the skin and strengthening the immunity system. The skin also feels smooth and soft.

How to use aloe vera as an antibiotic?

The primary method of using aloe vera as an antibiotic is by extracting its gel from the leaf. This gel needs to be applied directly to the affected area for best results.

For internal use, it is best to drink aloe vera juice everyday for a stronger immune system.

Ginger

Yes, ginger made the list too. For many, ginger is best known as a flavouring ingredient but it's time that you give this spice some credit for its healing properties. Ginger comes from a flowering plant and has been used as a medicine for many years. In Asia, people use it to treat sinus, cold and flu. But there's more to this under-rated spice. Ginger has been tested to have killed or treat some of the most dangerous cancer cells in the body. It has powerful anti-inflammatory and anti-bacterial properties that naturally destroy injurious bacteria. It is known to cure brain problems and even gut infections.

Health Benefits of Ginger:

Fights Against Fungal Infections – Ginger has strong anti-fungal properties that fight against fungal infections. They have been tested to treat these infections too.

Internal Ulcers – Yes ulcers can make their way into your stomach, intestines or other organs. Sometimes you may not even realize it's there. But don't worry. Regular consumption of ginger can greatly reduce your chances of getting any. And of course, In case you do develop an ulcer, you can treat it with ginger.

Diabetes – Ingesting ginger on the regular helps ward off diabetes as it helps maintain a normal blood sugar level.

Cancer – Studies have shown that ginger has the ability to fight cancerous cells such as lung, ovarian, breast, colon, pancreatic and skin cancers.

Gastric Problem – Regular stomach aches due to gastric trouble can be eased with ginger. While easing the pain caused by gastric, it also helps achieve a healthy bowel movement.

How to ingest ginger as an antibiotic?

Ginger can be added to your regular meal but of course it is most effective when consumed raw.

Ginger has a very bitter taste when eaten raw so add it to boiling water with one tablespoon honey to enhance its taste.

Adding shredded ginger to fruits or salad is not a bad idea.

Another way you can ingest it is by having ginger water. Simply add a few shredded pieces into boiling water and let it boil for a few minutes. Have this water once a day.

Rosemary

Rosemary is a natural antioxidant and helps decrease vascular permeability. It belongs to the mint family and is also known to have the ability to eliminate cancer cells. Rosemary is also a rich source if iron, calcium and vitamins. It is especially beneficial for people who suffer from mild asthma problems. It also has antimicrobials that help prevent and treat fungal infections by destroying harmful bacteria. These properties render this natural ingredient as one of the best ways to prevent yourself from the diseases which could pose serious harm to your health.

Health Benefits:

Healthy Immune System – Rosemary is known to possess antioxidants and anti-inflammatory compounds that help maintain a healthy immune system. It also naturally improves the body's blood circulation and helps the body to get rid of free radicals.

Strong Memory and Brain – Since it helps improve blood circulation, it also makes the body to function more efficiently by stimulating the memory and brain.

This is also because rosemary contains an antioxidant called carnosic acid that helps fight free radicals that are known to target the brain.

Cancer – Rosemary has anti-inflammatory and anti-tumor agent that help treat and prevents cancer cells.

Fight Infections – This aromatic plant also has anti-microbial properties to ward off fungi and bacteria to prevent infections.

Intestinal Ulcer – When suffering from inflammation or intestinal ulcer, a couple rosemary leaves would do the trick.

How to ingest rosemary as an antibiotic?

Rosemary acts as an essential herb in day to day cooking and if you don't use it regularly, perhaps you must start. Rosemary is available in two forms: fresh and dry. It can be consumed by adding a few leaves in your pasta, salad, fruits and your health drink.

Sage

Sage is another herb that serves as an excellent natural healing agent that is also high in anti-inflammatory compounds. Sage has been around for thousands of years and has been helping people heal and treat themselves naturally. This herb is great for mouth and throat problems such as tonsils, throat and mouth infections. When suffering from fever, cold and flu, sage works quicker than any other medicine. Needless to say, it is an essential and easily available immune booster and also balances the digestive system. Sage is widely used in medicines to treat digestive disorder and mental disorders too. White sage is known to be more effective than the regular sage when it comes to treating ailment.

Health Benefits:

Treating Alzheimer's – Using sage helps memory loss and other mental problems. It greatly helps people suffering from mild Alzheimer's problem by improving memory.

Diabetes – Occasional use of sage helps lower cholesterol and blood sugar.

How to ingest sage as an antibiotic?

There are a few methods of using sage to promote the health of the body:

Sage Tea: Add sage powder or finely chopped sage leaves in tea and let it boil for a few seconds. Strain and drink while it is hot. This is an excellent recipe for sore throat, throat infection and mouth infections as sage helps wipe out bacteria.

Sage Mouthwash: Add sage leaves to a water boiling pan and add a glass of water to it. Boil the water for a few minutes until the water extracts the fragrance and flavour of sage. Let the water sit for a few minutes. Use this water to gargle your mouth and throat. This works great if you are suffering from mouth or throat infection.

Sage Water: This is a great tonic to boost both, your energy and immunity. In a bowl mix together boiling water and sage leaves. Set it in place overnight. In the morning, strain the water and toss it in the refrigerator for a few hours. Transfer it into a sipper and drink your tonic all day.

Antiseptic Wash: Add lots of sage leaves to black tea and use this like an antiseptic liquid. You can pour it directly on a wound or cut to stop an infection and it also speeds the healing process.

Honey

Long before synthetic antibiotics came into picture, people used honey as a method to treat illnesses. Honey is believed to help maintain a healthy liver and also helps get rid of harmful toxins in the body. And since we are talking about antibiotic, honey is certainly loaded with antibacterial properties that treat bacteria naturally. Honey also contains active wound healing properties and antimicrobial that prevents certain bacteria from multiplying. Honey is widely used to treat wounds and cuts by forming a protective layer around the wound while creating a barrier against infection. It is extremely useful as it can be seen from the highlights of its useful properties. There are numerous benefits associated to this natural ingredient and it is used by large number of people for the positive effects it casts on the health.

Health Benefits:

Heals Wounds – Honey's antibacterial properties make it an excellent antiseptic agent. When applied on a fresh or infected wound, honey can soothe the skin while expediting the healing process.

Ulcers – Regular consumption of honey can heal stomach ulcers rapidly. It naturally promotes the growth of new and healthy tissue.

Burns and Infections – Bees make a protein that they transfer into honey and this protein helps treat burns and skin infections.

How to ingest honey as antibiotic?

Plain Honey: The best way to using honey when suffering from digestion or ulcer problems is by having a spoonful of plain honey.

Ginger Honey Tea: Ginger and honey tea works great when suffering from throat problem or indigestion. Add a few pieces of shredded ginger to hot black tea. Let it steep for a few minutes. Strain and add one tablespoon honey to the tea. Enjoy your healthy drink.

Cabbage

Cabbage belongs to the family of broccoli, kale and cauliflower. However between its family, cabbage is the only leafy vegetable that not only keeps you healthy but also disease-free. Some may also call it one of the world's healthiest foods. The number one reason to have cabbage is its sulphur compounds that helps combat cancer cells. It is also rich in Vitamin C which makes it a natural antibacterial agent.

Health Benefits:

Controlled Blood Pressure – Cabbage is rich in potassium which helps blood vessels to open up and regularize blood flow.

Healthy Immune System – Cabbage contains fibre and antibacterial property that strengthens the body's immune system. It is also rich in water which keeps the stomach healthy and prevents indigestion and constipation.

Low Risk of Heart Problems – The high content of polyphenol and anti-inflammatory compounds in cabbage prevents inflammation in the heart and also reduces the risk of heart disease.

Prevents Cancer – Many years of research has proved that people who consume cabbage have lower risk of developing cancer compared to the ones who don't eat this leafy vegetable. Cabbage contains a powerful cancer fighting compound called sulforaphane. It contains another compound called apigenin that helps fight tumors present in the form of breast cancer.

Healthy Brain – Red cabbage is loaded with vitamins and anthocyanins that prevent nerve damage and other mental disorders. These nutrients also help in boosting concentration and a healthy mental state.

Cabbage can be eaten raw, cooked or in form of juice. It should be a part of one's daily diet and here are a few ways you can add this ingredients to your regular meals.

Chop a couple raw cabbage leaves and garnish your soup with it. Mix well and eat.

You can also add shredded or chopped cabbage to your regular salad.

Take a few cabbage leaves and cut in medium size. Saute it slightly in butter. Add other vegetable if you like.

In a bowl, add shredded cabbage, garlic and olive oil. Mix well and enjoy.

Cinnamon

This famous spice has been treating people with its natural healing properties for many years. Cinnamon is commonly used by people who suffer from high blood sugar as cinnamon is known to lower blood sugar level. It contains antioxidants, anti-bacterial properties and helps reduce inflammation.

Health benefits:

Prevents Alzheimer's Disease – Studies have shown that cinnamon contains powerful compounds that can prevent Alzheimer's disease.

Treat/Prevents Multiple Sclerosis – Cinnamon prevents multiple sclerosis.

Treats Fungal Infection – Cinnamon contain a compound known as cinnamaldehyde that helps combat harmful bacteria and fungal infections.

Treat HIV Patients – A few strong agents present in cinnamon can treat yeast infection in HIV infected patients. Studies have also shown that cinnamon may be effective against HIV virus.

Controlled Blood Sugar in Diabetic Patients – People who suffer from high blood sugar can rely on cinnamon to control their blood sugar level naturally.

Throat Problem – Drinking cinnamon tea or water can soothe sore throats and other throat infections.

How to ingest honey as an antibiotic?

You can consume cinnamon by sprinkling cinnamon powder on cake or bread. This can also be added in other food during the cooking process.

Age old way of consuming cinnamon is by drinking cinnamon tea. Add cinnamon powder or cinnamon sticks in your tea. Have this tea once a day for effective results.

Basil

Basil is rich in various essential nutrients such as iron, potassium, vitamin A,K and C, magnesium and calcium. This herb is used as a seasoning ingredient in foods and offer much more than just its aromatic flavour. It has been around for several years but not many people are aware of its contribution towards a healthy body. Basil is known to treat many harmful bacterial infections even the most stubborn ones that have developed resistance against synthetic antibiotic drugs.

Health Benefits:

Boosts Immune System – Much like other herbs such as rosemary and sage, basil is also filled with antioxidants and anti-bacterial compounds that help fight against bacteria whilst strengthening the immune system.

Prevents Pre-Mature Aging – Powerful agents present in basil help fight against harmful molecules that prevent the heart, brain and liver from free radicals.

Strong Bones – Since basil is rich in Vitamin K, it promotes healthy and strong bones and prevents joint pains.

Controls Blood Pressure – Regular use of basil is beneficial for people who suffer from high blood pressure as potassium present in basil helps control blood pressure and heart rate.

How to ingest honey as an antibiotic?

There are many ways to eat fresh basil. One of the most common and popular is its use in pesto sauce.

You can also chop basil leaves and add them to fresh salad.

Final Words

Remember, these are natural methods to take care of your body. Regular consumption of these herbal antibiotics will help you stay healthy and away from harmful chemical induced medicines. But note that extreme of anything is bad for the body. So, take minimal dose of these herbal antibiotics and you should be good. Also, remember to consult your physician to find out if you are allergic to any ingredient.

Thank You Page

I want to personally thank you for reading my book. I hope you found information in this book useful and I would be very grateful if you could leave your honest review about this book. I certainly want to thank you in advance for doing this.

If you have the time, you can check my other books too.

www.ingramcontent.com/pod-product-compliance
Lightning Source LLC
LaVergne TN
LVHW021744060526
838200LV00052B/3458